Fuel for Success!

*You **can** lose weight,*
increase energy,
and live longer,
without hunger or misery!

Jill R. Johnson

Oxycise! International, Inc.
Littleton, CO

CAUTION!

The information contained in this book is not intended to replace medical consultation. The intent is only to offer health information to help you cooperate with your physician in your mutual quest for health. One should not participate in this exercise program, alter medications or change dietary habits except as advised by his or her physician.

Oxycise! International, Inc.
8170 S. University Blvd., #110
Littleton, CO 80122
(303)224-9588

http://www.oxycise.com

Contents

Chapter One

Listen
To Your Body

As a kid I remember watching my brothers play "gas station." They filled up my grandpa's gas tank with water from the garden hose and felt very mature with their assumption that anything they could pour in the gas tank would make the car run well. When my grandpa found out about the water in his gas tank you can be sure my brothers learned very quickly and permanently that although water has a very similar appearance and feel to gasoline, the car will not run on water. Even if the tank is totally full with water, you cannot drive it anywhere. Not only that, water in the gas tank will damage the engine.

What kind of food fuel are you putting into your body? Do you pay more attention to the fuel you put into your car than your body? I continue to be amazed at those I meet who are extremely careful about what products they use for their automobile and yet will literally put anything into their mouth that can fit down their throat.

If it's not your car you're concerned about, then it's your dog, cat, horse, bird, azaleas, roses, lawn, or garden. I see it all the time. Recently I was listening to a garden show on the radio. A woman called in totally distraught and with a trembling voice pled for the garden expert to help her get rid of an insect that was raiding her garden. She then described how she had placed lots of "sticky strips" to try and catch the bug. Then she had bought the recommended chemical spray, but it hadn't succeeded. Then she had heard from someone that if she washed the plants with soapy water the bugs would be killed. So this woman spent hours and hours, outside on her knees, washing the top and bottom of every single leaf on every single plant in her garden to try and keep them healthy.

My husband and I wandered through Oktoberfest at Vail, Colorado, this year with all of its featured bratwurst, knackwurst, and, of course, countless of varieties of German beer. We came upon a man who was heartily enjoying one of the large, fat, cholesterol-filled sausages while his dog sat patiently at his side. We commented in a sociable way, "Why don't you share some with your dog?" The man's very serious response was, "Oh, no, I can't do that. It's not good for him."

If you have been more concerned with the nutrition of something other than yourself, even if that other something is your children, then it's time to make a major paradigm shift. You will not be able to enjoy and/or take care of those other things, and they will not be able to enjoy you fully unless you take care of yourself first. This does not mean you should become obsessed with yourself and neglect everything else. But if you have neglected yourself for years, you may need to invest in yourself for awhile.

Remember that your body is more complicated in structure and function than your car. If you were to put water in your car's gas tank, it might mess up your engine, but a lot of the car wouldn't be directly affected — the wheels, body, interior, etc. But when you put damaging fuel into your body, every cell is affected — your brain, heart, lungs, all vital organs, skin, nerves, eyes, digestive tract . . . you get the picture. When you put the right fuel in your body, imagine the consequences: Every cell is affected!!! You have a healthy vibrant body from the *inside out*!

Affluence and its follies.

Food is strange. It seems to be only in times of affluence that humans develop such a strange relationship with food. Food is used to show love, power, prosperity, and passion. "Pigging out" is considered entertainment. We have feasts and food festivals for every excuse anyone can think of. Some of the most damaging things we can put in our bodies are considered "treats" rather than the poison they really are.

In a car and in other mechanical engines the tank overflows if you put in too much fuel. If you put in the wrong kind of fuel, the engine won't work. Can you imagine standing there at a gas station pumping gas into the gas tank until it is full and then continuing to stand there with it overflowing because your car "really likes" that kind of gas? Maybe you let it overflow because you don't know when you'll be able to fill up again. Have you ever overfilled your gas tank because that's your car's favorite kind of gas? Or how about putting gas into the oil pan and oil into the gas tank, because you like variety?

The reasons for overfeeding or using the wrong fuel sound facetious when applied to auto maintenance, but somehow those same attitudes are accepted when applied to fuel for humans. What does it take for humans to consider food as a fuel for the body rather than a substance that only has to pass the taste bud test? Obviously obesity, illness, and death haven't convinced most people yet. Besides there are always Tums, Rolaids, Tagamet, Ex Lax, Pepto-bismol, and Kaopectate. And then, of course, there are good health insurance plans available with great disability and death benefits.

You are different. You are seeking the truth and trying to do the best you can for your body. You've learned about the number one fuel which is oxygen, and have been utilizing it more fully with Oxycise! Your body also needs clean-burning food. Food is not only necessary, it is good. But it seems that with every good thing on earth, it can be distorted into something damaging — even dangerous. Food, which is meant to be fuel for health and life-giving, has become one of the biggest killers in America. In this chapter you will learn simple food principles that will give a tremendous boost to your weight loss goals, and balance and vitality to your life.

Listen to your body.

A client sent the following diet to me with this note: "I have followed this diet religiously for a long time. Perhaps others do as well."

Stress Diet

Breakfast
½ grapefruit
a slice whole-wheat bread
8 ounces skim milk

Lunch
4 ounces broiled chicken breast
1 cup steamed zucchini
1 Oreo cookie
1 cup herb tea

Mid-afternoon Snack
Rest of package of Oreo cookies
1 quart Rocky Road ice cream
1 jar hot fudge sauce

I admit it. I have followed that kind of diet more times than I care to remember. But it has been many years ago and I have confidence that I will never do it again. Why? Because I have learned to listen to my body. If you truly want to gain freedom from obesity then you will need to learn to listen too. The main concept that permeates every aspect of the Oxycise! lifestyle is that you have the power to master your body from the inside out.

When we were little, our parents told us when and what to eat. We also learned that if we cleaned our plate we were helping all the starving children in Africa or wherever children were starving at the time. I personally helped many starving children and cleaned my plate many times. My husband once challenged his dad who was telling him about all the starving children in China by saying, "Name three." He was sent away from the table. From then on he learned to clean his plate. As his awareness of the world increased, so did his sense of civic duty, and he took even more helpings of food so he could help even more starving children. He currently feels that there are innumerable Chinese who are indebted to him.

As we watched cartoons and children's shows on TV, we didn't see dancing heads of lettuce or singing broccoli encouraging us to buy them and eat them. In fact, in my 40 years of watching TV, I don't ever remember any ads for fruits or vegetables.

Likewise when we went to the grocery store with our moms and stood in the check-out line, what was within our reach?? Gum, candy bars, packages of donuts! There weren't (and still aren't) any last minute, impulse buying, encouragements to be sure and take home fresh carrots or whole grain bread. And speaking of bread, there seemed to be a conspiracy while I was growing up to see who could make bread with the least amount of natural ingredients and to see how far wheat could be distorted from its natural state. Bread nearly turned into cake.

The external pressures continue. Just look at a typical evening of commercials on TV, or billboards on the freeway.

- Serious testimonials convince you that Snicker's candy bars can help you through the day.
- Pizza smothered in fat (called cheese, sausage, pepperoni) is supposed to make you hungry.
- Arch Deluxe (another name for fat).

- Biggie Fries. (Why are advertising campaigns that appeal to a gluttonous nature so successful?)
- Alcohol and tobacco products have their own deceitful promotions.
- Plop, plop, fizz, fizz . . . just take a pill to rid yourself of any discomfort.

All of these ads and the scenarios described earlier overwhelmingly draw your attention to external stimuli. None of them gives you any encouragement to listen to or follow your body's true signals and messages. Can you imagine an ad encouraging you to eat healthy foods so you don't feel the need to buy antacids? You are pressured constantly to have your taste buds guide your decisions and your life. Or you are doing what you feel required to do, whether your body needs it or not. The tragic result is that you are no longer listening to your body and hence are not enjoying the optimum health you deserve.

It is extremely difficult to listen to your body in our society. We're always in a hurry, and we're often surrounded by so many other voices, including the overbearing voice of immediate gratification. In addition we have traditions such as big breakfasts, Valentine candy, and Thanksgiving dinners, that aren't considered successful unless no one can move afterwards.

Many of you have read about or have been to workshops on choosing to be *proactive* rather than *reactive* in your business or relationships. Stephen R. Covey, in his extraordinary book *The 7 Habits of Highly Effective People*, identifies as Habit #1: Be Proactive.

"Our basic nature is to act, and not be acted upon. As well as enabling us to choose our response to particular circumstances, this empowers us to create circumstances. . . to take initiative. It means that as human beings, we are responsible for our own lives. Look at the word *responsibility* — "response-ability" — the ability to choose your response.

"Proactivity is part of human nature, and, although the proactive muscles may be dormant, they are there . . . . If you wait to be acted upon, you *will* be acted upon.

"The difference between people who exercise initiative and those who don't is literally the difference between night and day. I'm not talking about a 25 to 50 percent difference in effectiveness; I'm talking about a 5,000-plus percent difference."

Those same principles apply here. If you respond to external messages with your food choices you are being *reactive*. You are reacting to whatever external stimuli comes along. If you listen and act upon the internal messages your body sends, then you are *proactive* and choosing what's truly best for you.

Read through the following examples of external and internal messages.

External Messages

It's 6:00. Time for dinner.
Clean your plate or you can't go out and play.
We won the game. Let's celebrate.
The buffet is "All You Can Eat" so I better load up.
Singing chocolate candies on TV.

It's my birthday. I should indulge myself.
You had a rough day. Here's a box of chocolates.
What will the host think if I don't eat the prime rib?
Starving yourself to lose weight.
Using appetite suppressants to curb your appetite.
Being swayed by advertising when shopping.
My whole family is fat so it must be genetic.

Internal Messages

I'm not hungry right now.
I'd love a nice, cold drink of juice.
I really am thirsty.
I really am hungry.
I'm full.
I've had enough.
I only need a little bit.
When I eat this, I feel energized.
Vegetables would taste great.
Shopping with nutrition in mind.
There's nothing on the menu that would
feel good in my body.
I choose to be slim and healthy.

Which kind of messages do you regularly respond to? If you find that you primarily live your life by reacting to the external messages, then stop. There are so many food plans, diet programs, and appetite suppressants out there it makes your head swim. You feel like curling up with your Twinkies and Coke for comfort from the barrage of messages coming your way. Most of them make me angry. Your body is not a machine and does not need chemicals poured into it to function. I also don't believe that humans can only be healthy if they weigh and measure their food either.

I do believe that if you listen, really listen, to your body, it will guide you. Listening is critical to taking care of yourself. You do have an inner voice that inherently knows what is right and good for you. As you fuel your body, take the time to listen to it.

For the next day, watch for all the food and body messages around you. How often do you *react* to the external messages? How often do you *act* upon the internal messages? If the food principles I teach you are new, apply them for a full month, then listen to your body and see what it has to say. I'll bet you dollars to sugar and fat-free doughnuts that it will holler a big, resounding, "THANK YOU!" Also, as you continue to act upon your internal messages you will, just as Covey describes, experience a 5,000-plus percent increase in effectiveness.

Do not undereat. Do not overeat.

Listen to your body. Listen to your body.

Do not undereat. Do not overeat.

Listen to your body. Listen to your body.

Chapter Two

Your
Food G.P.A.

Counting fat grams and calories . . . measuring portions and servings . . . deciphering labels . . . . You need to be a rocket scientist to follow all the nutrition advice being fired at you these days. What I am about to present to you is a simplified approach to healthy eating. I've simply given quality "grades" to different foods according to their benefit for weight loss and general health, just as you receive scores on papers in school. Simply average your grades each day to track your progress.

You'll like this system because you don't have to be perfect to achieve success. I want you to get rid of those deep, inbred notions of "cheating." Just yank them out from all those dark places. You don't need to be guilt-laden anymore about what you eat. Misery in any form is not part of the Oxycise! lifestyle.

You will feel so good and have so much energy with this nutrition that making healthy choices will become second nature to you.

- You will LOSE WEIGHT and maintain a healthy body size.

- Your taste buds will delight in the taste of fresh food.

- Your entire body will function so much better, you'll be angry that you wasted so much time in poor health when a few simple changes made all the difference.

- Your digestive and elimination systems will function smoothly.

- No more R-O-L-A-I-D-S, because you don't need relief.

- You will feel vibrant.

After eating this way for a few weeks, you will be amazed that you ever craved some of the food you used to snarf down.

"Better than" philosophy.

You are not a robot, so you have to learn to live in the world of choices and decisions, especially with what you eat. Modern transportation and refrigeration provide endless possibilities . . . so does progress with chemicals and synthesized food.

Everything doesn't have to be treated as sterile or black and white. But if you have a general idea of what reaction your body will have with different food products, you can make better choices.

I've created a grading scale in accordance with what I've found to work successfully in real life — not just in a laboratory setting. You are subject to moods, peer pressure, media advertising, etc. If you understand how food works in your body, you can make "better than" choices when faced with a grocery store full of selections. For instance, for many years dieters have been drinking diet soda because it has little or no calories. Please look at the food lists. Diet soda rates an "F" because it, as well as regular soda, wreaks havoc in your body due to its high phosphoric acid, artificial sweetners, and other chemical content. However, fresh fruit juice rates an "A" regardless of calories. Fresh fruit juice is "better than" any kind of soda. Please switch to choosing what is better for your body.

Straight A's for weight loss.

Take a few minutes now to look over the food lists. Every food available is not listed — especially the packaged kind. To grade a food not listed, simply identify what its characteristics are and grade it by comparison to the foods already on the lists using your good judgment. If you choose packaged food, you'll need to read the ingredients and then grade it. The recipe/meal ideas are very quick and simple suggestions for every day eating. There are many good low-fat vegetarian cookbooks available to help you plan more meals.

Don't get upset if your favorite food is an "F." The foods on the "F" list will never aid you in keeping your body slim and they don't promote good health. But if you insist on keeping some of those foods in your life, here's all you do:

1. Eat these items very infrequently. If you eat nine "A" items in a day and one "F" item, that will average out to a "B" for the day. If your weekly average is six "A" days and one "B" day, then you still have an "A" average for the week and are doing great things for your body.

2. Learn to properly combine food as described in Chapter Four.

3. On the rare occasions when you do eat one of these items, listen to how your body feels afterwards. The sluggishness, discomfort, and even pain are reminders that you are doing something damaging to your body. Is the momentary taste worth the long-term damage?

My ratings may be different than your hired dietician. There may be someone somewhere, who has successfully lost permanent weight through the advice of a professional dietician or nutritionist, but I personally don't know of anyone. My lists are based on the most current nutritional and health information available combined with a little bit of realism — so you *can* live in our culture and attend an occasional birthday or office party without getting psychologically involved with the food.

It's time to start!

You won't need to record your food intake for your entire life, but while you are making changes and developing new habits it is important to write down what you are doing. This way you are accountable to yourself. It will also help you identify the problem if you aren't achieving the success you desire. Before you know it, you will be listening to your body and responding to its real needs and the lists will become superfluous.

1.   *List food items and their grade as you eat them during the day. Do not record detailed amounts.*

Example:

cantaloupe	A
orange juice	A
banana	A
strawberries	A
carrots	A
peas	A
broccoli	A

Or just:

fruit	A
veggies	A

2.   *Don't worry about listing spices, condiments, and misc.*

3.   Assign points for food from the different lists.

Food List Grade	Points Given	Average
A	4	3.4 - 4.0
B	3	2.7 - 3.3
C	2	1.9 - 2.6
D	1	1.0 - 1.8
F	0	0.0 - 0.9

4.   Average your grade for the day.

Example:

1.	fruit	4
2.	fruit	4
3.	juice	4
4.	fruit smoothie	4
5.	veggie soup	4
6.	croutons	3
7.	bagel	3
8.	w/ veggies	4
9.	frozen fruit bar	4
10.	baked potato	4
11.	salad	4
12	sesame seeds	3
13.	banana	4

TOTAL POINTS   49

Total Points   ÷   Number of Items   =   Daily Average

Example:

49 Points ÷ 13 Items = 3.77 Daily Average

An "A" for the day!

5.   *Give yourself a sticker for doing such a good job.*

Always give yourself credit for your accomplishments. Changing years of habit takes substantial effort, so go ahead and pat yourself on the back.

6.   *At the end of each week average your daily grades to find your weekly average.*

Example:

Sunday	4
Monday	4
Tuesday	3
Wednesday	4
Thursday	4
Friday	4
Saturday	3
TOTAL POINTS	26

26 ÷ 7 = 3.71

Weekly Average 3.71

An "A" for the week!

7.   *As you fuel your body day after day, keep track of your G.P.A. and you will be able to see and feel which of the following categories you fit in:*

G.P.A.	Weight and Health Category
A average	Healthy weight loss if needed and great health.
B average	General maintenance and good health.
C average	Average health, at possible risk for health and weight problems.
D average	If you don't have good health insurance, better get it now.
F average	Make sure your will is in order.

Chapter 3

Three Day
Oxycise! Cleanse

Spring cleaning the easy way.

You want success. You want a great body. You want a healthy body. So why do you have so much junk food and unhealthy food sitting around in your home and office? Get rid of it! If you can't stand to throw it away then give it away. Don't give to anyone you care about — you don't want to contribute to destroying their health.

It's simple. Start in your kitchen pantry, shelves and drawers. Clean out the refrigerator and freezer. Get rid of garbage food that's in your desk at work. Just do it.

Get your body ready for success.

Now it's time to start cleaning out the rotten, impacted garbage inside your body. More than likely, you have quite a few years of dumping anything in sight into your body and before you can begin to function at your optimum level, you need to clean it out. Cleaning your body is a lot easier than cleaning the garage or attic and it's a lot more fun. I've seen many different cleanses promoted — most of them with complicated directions. Mine is simple.

The Three-Day Oxycise! Cleanse

If oxygen in every cell makes such a difference in fat burning and health, eating oxygen-rich food will bring you even more exciting results.

For the next three days, fuel your body with only fruits and vegetables. *Any* fruits and vegetables. Just walk up and down the produce section of your grocery store and let your imagination soar. On occasion I have heard people complain that produce is so expensive. That excuse always floors me. Compare the price of a grocery cart full of produce to a grocery cart full of meat, seafood, chips, dip, pop, candy, cigarettes, beer, etc.

Guidelines:

1.   **Eat anything on the A list.**

- Prepare food any way you like — fresh, baked, boiled, steamed, blended, or microwaved.
- Use any herbs or spices desired.
- You may use salad dressings.

2. **Use fresh produce as much as possible.**

    - Frozen (unsweetened, and without sauces) is your next best choice.
    - Dried fruits and vegetables are good.
    - Canned is less desirable but okay (be sure it doesn't have added sugars or sauces).

3. **Fresh vegetable and fruit juices are wonderful.**

    - Frozen juice is good (be sure it is pure juice, without corn syrup or other added sugars).
    - Canned 100% juice is fine, too.

4. **Eat any time of day.**

5. **Eat any amount.**

6. **Do not go hungry.**

7. **Eat a variety of food.**

    - There is no single "magic" food.

8. **Listen to what your body needs.**

Warning, warning . . .

A word of warning. If eating fruits and vegetables is a whole new experience for you, your body may react at first. It is kind of like a child fussing because you're making him take his medicine. You may experience stomach cramps or pains as your intestines are cleansed of all the undigested matter that has been accumulating there. Consider it a small price to pay for the years of abuse you've already put your body through. The discomfort, if you have any at all, will pass in a day or so.

Get in touch with your body.

That's all there is to the Oxycise! Cleanse. It truly is simple. Your body will respond immediately to good treatment. Your taste buds will be refreshed and begin to crave clean, wholesome food. Your digestive system will be flushed out and ready for healthy action. But one of the most important results of the Oxycise! Cleanse is that your mind will start to recognize and respond to your internal body messages. These messages have always been there and now you are "in tune" enough to hear them. Don't ever lose touch with this ability and you will have an important, even essential tool available to you for the rest of your life as you continue to improve your health.

Chapter 4

Food for Life!
A Week by Week Plan
for Weight Loss and Health

Week #1 for Weight Loss and Health

You've completed the *Three-Day Oxycise! Cleanse.* Congratulations! I bet you feel great, not only because you've been eating such wonderful food, but because you are well on your way to achieving the body you desire.

Keep eating all the food from the "A" List to your heart's delight. You are a live person. Remember to eat living, fresh food as much as possible, full of vitamins and active enzymes.

Add the "B" List.

Now you will add the items on the "B" List to your food plan. These few items are essential for a lifetime of health. Besides the health benefits, they taste great, add a lot of variety to your menu, and feel good in your body.

Complex carbohydrates.

Certain foods listed on the "A" and "B" Lists are known as complex carbohydrates. Potatoes, grains, and rice, which I have placed on the "B" List, fit into this category. Pasta and bread, which are on the "C" List, are complex carbohydrates, yet are processed farther and hence, have a little different reaction in your body.

Complex carbohydrate is just a fancy name for those great foods that your body thrives on. These foods are especially effective for weight loss because they have been shown to have what has been termed as a "negative calorie effect" because your body actually uses more energy/calories to utilize these particular foods than are in the food in the first place. Some of you may still have the mind set that you will gain weight by eating starches like potatoes or rice. Not so! All the fat and grease that is frequently loaded onto these foods can ruin your body, but not these foods by themselves. In fact, if you want to have a great weight-loss day, eat two or three potatoes along with any food from the "A" List, and you will feel and see the difference.

Eat what you need.

Foods on the "B" List will need to be processed and cooked to some degree. You don't have to count servings. Just eat what your body needs. On different days you may feel differently, so don't worry about making each day the same. Just as you use different amounts of gas in your car on different days depending on the amount of travel or type of terrain, so does your body need different amounts of fuel on different days. If you can train your mind to quit consciously giving eating directions, your body will let you know when it is full or empty and even what kind of food it needs. At first you will have to make efforts retraining your system, but it won't be long before it takes care of itself, and all your food choices will become second nature.

Eating late at night promotes weight gain.

The time you eat food *does* make a difference in your body. Your metabolism slows down naturally at night. Your digestive system is busy processing your fuel intake from the day. Everything about your body is getting ready for sleep. Research has shown that eating your food early in the day promotes weight loss, while eating the exact same food late in the evening promotes weight gain.

Now if it's 8 p.m. and you think you're going to die, don't go out for ice cream. Have a piece of fruit or snack from the "A" List or some hash browns (cooked without oil , in a non-stick pan). Or mix up a fruit drink with orange juice, bananas, and strawberries. Make it nice and thick — ooh that sounds good.

Fruit keeps your morning "smooth."

Fruit has a cleansing effect and will clear impacted matter from your intestinal walls and flush it out of your system in the form of loose stools. By eliminating these toxins every morning, you will feel energetic and ready for work, play, and Oxycise!

Abundance mentality.

Now that you have the right road map, your attitude will make a big difference. This is the time to focus on developing an Abundance Mentality:

> "There is so much I'm achieving by eating this way."

> "I am in a better position to help others by taking care of myself."

> "My friends and family are my allies in making these changes."

> "I am worth taking the time to learn these new and healthy skills."

Benefits.

By eating these foods you will be amazed at how great you feel. You will not feel tired and heavy after lunch. Your day will be more productive. *And* your body will be operating on clean fuel so that as you Oxycise! you will experience even more weight loss and health benefits. By the way, have your cholesterol and blood pressure checked in a month. You and your doctor may just be shocked at the improvement.

Week #2 for Weight Loss and Health

You've completed the *Three-Day Oxycise! Cleanse* and *Week #1 for Weight Loss and Health*. Your body is starting to wonder if it can depend on such wonderful nutrients coming to it on a consistent basis. It's wondering if is should lower its set point mechanism. Be consistent with Oxycise! and with the Fuel for Success nutrition and I guarantee that your set point will plunge downward.

Add the "C" List.

So far, by mainly eating from the "A" List and occasionally from the "B" List, you are easily able to maintain an "A" average for your personal Food G.P.A. This week you may add foods from the "C" List. Be aware that if you use too many "C" foods, you will move to a "B" or "C" average. This works fine for general health and maintenance, but if weight loss is your goal, then you will want to keep an "A" average and only use the "C" List a few times a week. Be sure to keep eating lots and lots of live, fresh, oxygen-rich food.

Week #3 for Weight Loss and Health

How are you feeling these days? I know that if you are faithfully doing Oxycise! at least 5 times a week, and if you are maintaining an "A" average with your Food G.P.A. then you are seeing and feeling a difference in your body. Doesn't it feel great? It's a wonderful experience to master your body from the inside out.

Habits: You choose your orbit.

All of you who own a television have watched with a certain sense of awe as rocket engines were ignited and enough force was created to blast space shuttles from the tremendous gravity pull of the earth and send them into orbit. More preparation, focus, and energy were spent on the first few minutes and first few miles of travel than were used over the next several million miles.

Your current body habits also have a tremendous gravity pull. You know you need to do something to change your body. This book teaches you what to do. But you have to *want* to do these things in order to develop the habit."Lifting off" from years of traditions, false information, and unhealthy habits will take a big chunk of effort. But you will soon be launched into a healthy orbit as Oxycise! and eating well become your permanent habit and tradition.

Allow yourself a month or more to establish your new eating habits. You are blasting off on a powerful and rewarding program. Give it every chance for success. Keep looking forward to the abundant benefits for you and others. As you break out of the gravity pull of your former unhealthy habits, your real freedoms will take on whole new dimensions. You are going to love your body!

You decide your lifestyle.

At this point you have some decisions to make concerning the rate at which you want to change your body. For these first several weeks I have been holding your hand and telling you exactly what to do. Hopefully you can feel and see the difference in your body, which will motivate you to make healthy decisions on your own now. To aid you in this, I have listed some guidelines which demonstrate how your actions will determine your rate of weight loss. There is no law that says you have to make a body change quickly. You have the freedom to make that decision. You may decide to "take the bull by the horns" and get rid of fat as quickly as possible, or you may decide to achieve your goals more gradually. Any point along the scale is just fine, as long as you are being true to yourself and living a healthy lifestyle.

Lifestyle Guidelines

Dramatic weight loss.

1. Oxycise! every single day.
   Do at least 30 repetitions. For even more dramatic results, Oxycise! twice a day. Also, take advantage of any free moments when you can do a few extra reps while waiting — at a red light, for an elevator, for water to boil, for the microwave, etc.

2. Eat only fresh fruit, fruit juices, and drinks from the "A" list in the early morning.

3. Eat the bulk of your fuel needs from both the "A" and "B" Lists from late morning until about 6 p.m.

4. After 6 p.m. keep your fuel intake very low and eat only "A" foods. If you work a night shift, adjust these times in accordance with your sleep patterns.

Good, steady weight loss.

1. Oxycise! at least five times per week. Fit in several "extra" reps during the day.

2. Use the "A" and "B" foods most of the time.

3. Follow the food-combining guidelines.

4. Maintain an "A" average using foods from any lists.

Slower, more gradual weight loss.

1. Oxycise! four or five times per week. Fit in extra reps during the day.

2. Follow the food-combining guidelines.

3. Maintain a "B+" average using foods from any lists.

General health and body maintenance.

1. Oxycise! three times per week or do fewer reps four or five times per week. Fit in extra reps during the day.

2. Follow the food-combining guidelines.

3. Maintain a "B" average using foods from any lists.

NO weight loss or health benefits.

1. Make no effort to increase your oxygen consumption.

2. Put anything into your body you can swallow.

Chapter Five

Food Lists

for

Your Food G.P.A.

"A" FOODS

Eat lots and lots of produce. Use oxygen-rich, fresh produce as much as possible. Be sure processed produce has no added salt, sugar of any kind, or chemicals.

Rating scale for fruits, vegetables and juices.

> Best: fresh, raw
> Better: frozen
> Good: dried
> Okay: canned

The following food lists are not all-inclusive. They are meant to give you an idea of what to eat during your Oxycise! cleanse, as well as to illustrate the enormous variety of wonderful food available to delight your palate and bring health to your body. Always avoid any food or spice that causes an allergic reaction or other problem. Be sure to have a variety of fruits, vegetables and juices. Be creative!

FRUITS

apple
apple juice or cider
applesauce, unsweetened
apricots
banana
berries, all kinds
cantaloupe
carambola

cherimoya
cherries
cranberries, unsweetened
crenshaw melon
dates
figs, fresh, dried
fruit juice concentrate
fruit cocktail, no added sugar
grape juice
grapefruit
grapefruit juice
grapes
guava
honeydew melon
kiwi
kumquat
lemon juice
lime juice
loquat
lychee
mandarin oranges
mango
nectarine
orange
orange juice
papaya
passion fruit
passion fruit, juice
peach
pear
persimmon
pineapple
plums

pomegranate
prunes, fresh, dried, juice
pummelo
quince
raisins
strawberries
tangelos
tangerine
watermelon

VEGETABLES

artichoke
arugula
asparagus
avocado
beans, all kinds
beets
bok choy
broccoli
brussels sprouts
burdock
cabbage
carrots
cauliflower
celery root
celery
chicory
chilies
chives
cilantro
collard greens
coriander

corn
cucumber
eggplant
endive
escarole
greens: beet, collard, chard
Jerusalem artichoke
jicama
kale
kohlrabi
leeks
lentils
lettuce, all kinds
lima beans
mint
mushrooms
okra
olives
onions, all types
parsley
parsnips
pea pods, Chinese
peas, all kinds
peppers, all kinds
pimento
radishes
rhubarb
rutabaga
salsify
seaweed
shallots
spinach
sprouts (alfalfa, lentil, mung bean, wheat)

squash, all kinds
sweet potatoes
Swiss chard
taro root
tomato juice
tomatoes, fresh, paste, sauce, puree, stewed
vegetable juice
water chestnuts
watercress
yams

SPICES, CONDIMENTS, AND MISCELLANEOUS

barbecue sauces, no oil
garlic
ginger
horseradish
hot pepper sauces
ketchup, low sodium
lemon or lime juice, fresh or bottled
lemon pepper
Mrs. Dash
mustard
onions
parsley
pepper
salt

> Use salt sparingly. Don't cook with it. If you don't use packaged and processed foods, you will probably not need to be concerned that you're using too much salt. If you have high blood pressure, kidney problems, or swelling, then follow your physician's advice.

soy sauce

spices, all kinds
steak sauce
Tabasco

SAUCES AND DRESSINGS

bouillon
   Avoid bouillon if you need to restrict your sodium intake
marinara and spaghetti sauces
   Either make your own or purchase bottled sauces that are
   made totally from vegetables.
picante sauce
salsa
vinegar, all kinds
salad dressings*
   Chemical-free, any kind
   Homemade dressings are great!

My philosophy is this:

- Eat lots of live, fresh produce.

- Use any kind of dressing . . . just don't have the
  lettuce leaves floating in it.

- If you're perfectly happy with oil-free, sugar-free,
  dairy-free, chemical-free dressings and you eat
  lots of main-dish salads, then that's great! But for
  many people, just having the freedom to use any
  salad dressing suddenly opens up new doorways
  to health because they start eating so much more
  oxygen-filled, fresh food.

*This is an area in which I differ with many health gurus. Salad dressings have gotten such a bad "rap" due to their high amount of fat that many of you are afraid to use them. What I've seen happen in real life is that people quit eating salads because they taste so empty without a good dressing. But because your bodies crave the vitamins, minerals, and crunchy texture that you're missing, you end up eating all kinds of poor quality food instead.

**Special note: I have observed that many people are able to make healthy eating a lifetime choice instead of a one-week deprivation exercise simply by using salad dressings.

SNACKS

baked tortilla chips (Tostitos or other brand with no added fat)
dried fruit
finger veggies
    Try baby carrots, cherry tomatoes, broccoli, cauliflower, or celery.
fresh fruit, any fruit
frozen fruit bars, 100% fruit, no added sugar
fruit smoothie
fruit bars, 100% fruit, no added sugar
fruit leather
instant vegetable soups
pickles
popcorn, air popped, no oil or butter
    Try sprinkling garlic, chili, curry, onion powder, creole seasoning, or sprinkle soy sauce or water on it and sprinkle with brewer's yeast.

raisins
salsa
sorbet, made from fruit and fruit juice only

DRINKS

fruit juices, hot or cold
herbal teas
mineral water
noncaffeinated hot drinks
    Sipp, Pero, Kaffree Roma, Cafix, Postum
tea, noncaffeinated
vegetable juices, hot or cold
water, my personal favorite

EASY RECIPE AND MEAL IDEAS

Fruit Smoothies
My family loves these in the morning or on a hot day.
    Mix the following in a blender:
        4 ice cubes in a blender
        1 cup of orange juice
        1 banana

    Add any other fresh or frozen fruit you desire —
strawberries, peaches, blueberries, etc.

Totally Veggie Spaghetti
    1 spághetti squash, baked or microwaved
    marinara sauce or spaghetti sauce

Shred the inside of spaghetti squash onto a plate to look like
noodles. Pour sauce on top. Enjoy!

Tostada

Layer your favorite ingredients on baked tortilla chips.

> beans
> olives
> onions
> tomatoes
> jalapeno peppers
> shredded lettuce
> avocado
> salsa

Veggie Stew

Slice or dice vegetables. Cook until tender in any flavor bouillon or vegetable juice.

> carrots
> onions
> squash
> mushrooms
> beans
> corn

Main Dish Salad

> lettuce, romaine, green leaf, and/or other kinds
> carrots, sliced or shredded
> purple onion, diced
> mushrooms, sliced
> cucumbers, sliced
> tomatoes, wedged
> sprouts, any variety
> beans, any kind
> green peppers

Toss together these and any other fresh ingredients. Serve with salad dressing.

Other ideas:

Vegetarian Shish Kabobs
Vegetarian Baked Beans
Lentil Soup
Split Pea Soup
Black Bean Soup
Fruit Salad
Fruit Soup
Corn on the Cob
Curried Vegetables

Mmm! It all makes my mouth water!

B" FOODS

barley
couscous
grains
    buckwheat
    cracked wheat
    grits
    rolled oats
    triticale
    whole wheat
potatoes, all kinds
    frozen varieties, no added oil
    instant mashed
    new
    red
    russet
    white
rice, all kinds
    basmati
    brown
    instant, this is less desirable but okay
    long grain
    mixes
        Rice-a-Roni and other brands (Follow directions but leave out the butter.)
    wild
vegetarian burgers
    Be sure to read the label.
    Cook without oil.

SPICES, CONDIMENTS, AND MISCELLANEOUS

nonstick cooking spray
nonfat mayonnaise

SAUCES AND DRESSINGS

stir-fry sauce
teriyaki sauce
low-fat soymilk, use only on cereal, not for a drink

SNACKS

baked potato chips
rice cakes
baked french fries
instant oatmeal
canned beans
instant soups with vegetables and rice or potatoes
instant mashed potatoes

EASY RECIPE AND MEAL IDEAS

Modify any of your favorite recipes by removing the oil, fat, sugar, and meat. You'll come up with lots of delicious ideas.

Baked Potato With Salad Bar
Bake or microwave a large potato. Slice open. Pile on all sorts of salad fixings like red leaf lettuce, cucumbers, mushrooms, onions, carrots, sprouts, etc. Top with dressing.

Baked Potato With Soy Sauce
Top a baked potato with soy sauce. Try it, you'll like it.

Hash Brown Potatoes

Shred fresh potatoes with a food processor or grater, or use frozen hash browns with no added grease or oil. Cook in a nonstick skillet until browned. Top with ketchup, if desired.

Optional: Add diced onions, shredded carrots, or other chopped vegetables.

Skillet Potatoes

Slice fresh potatoes and brown in nonstick skillet. Add onions, if desired.

French Fries

Slice and bake your own. Sprinkle with any spices or seasonings.

Rice and Beans

Prepare any kind of rice. Top with any kind of beans. Smother with green chiles or salsa.

Rice and Spinach

Prepare any kind of rice. Cook fresh or frozen spinach. Mix together and sprinkle on lemon juice or vinegar.

Stir Fry

Saute your favorite veggies in water. Add stir-fry sauce. Serve over rice.

Whole Wheat Chili

Soak wheat overnight, then boil until tender. Add to your favorite vegetarian chili recipe.

Hot Cereal
    Whole wheat, oatmeal, grits, cream of wheat, etc. Top with cinnamon, strawberries, bananas, peaches, raisins, etc. Do not use milk. You may use low-fat soymilk if desired.

Other ideas:

Mashed Potatoes
Potato, Rice, or Barley and Vegetable Soup
Spanish Rice
Curried Rice and Vegetables

"C" FOODS

bagels
bread
    whole wheat
    rye
    sourdough
    french
    white, less desirable, but okay
bread sticks
cereal
    Choose those that have as their main ingredients: whole wheat, oats, oat bran, brown rice, corn, barley. Avoid those with added oils and sugars.
cornmeal
    cornbread
    polenta
crackers, baked, fat-free
croutons, fat-free
English muffins
hummus
Melba toast
muffins, fat-free, sweetened with fruit juice
noodles and pasta, all kinds
    angel hair
    fettucine
    lasagna
    linguine
    macaroni
    ramen
    shell
    soba

spaghetti
spinach
tomato basil
whole wheat
nuts, raw, all kinds
> All nuts should be eaten raw. They contain high quality nutrition and are used well by the human system.
> Never eat roasted nuts. Avoid overeating nuts.

pancakes
pita bread
quick breads (banana, pumpkin, cornbread, etc.)
> fat-free, no added sugar

rolls, all kinds
seeds, raw, all kinds
> Follow the same guidelines as nuts.

tofu, use sparingly as it is high in fat
tortillas, nonfat
TVP (textured vegetable protein)
waffles

SPICES, CONDIMENTS, AND MISCELLANEOUS

baking powder
baking soda
use applesauce instead of oil for baking
> measure equal amounts

use egg replacer for baking

SAUCES AND DRESSINGS

jam, pure fruit, no sugar
honey
syrup, maple or fruit

SNACKS

bagel with honey
baked bagel chips
crackers, baked
English muffin with 100% fruit jam
fig bars
leftovers from dinner
packaged cookies, made without fat and using fruit juice for
    sweetening
pretzels
granola bars, low-fat

EASY RECIPE AND MEAL IDEAS

Veggie Sandwich
Use any variety of bread, roll, bagel, or pita. Fill with
tomatoes, cucumbers, carrots, mushrooms, onions,
lettuce, sprouts, peppers, mustard, or vinegar.
Delicious!

Waffle, Pancake, French Toast
Cook without oil. Use egg replacer. Top with syrup,
honey, or fruit jam.

Potato Salad
Use nonfat mayonnaise as you combine ingredients for
your favorite potato salad.

Veggie Tacos
Fill soft flour tortillas with any of the following: beans,
rice, peppers, chiles, onions, carrots, broccoli, sprouts,
salsa.

Pasta Salad

Prepare pasta of your choice. Add vegetables of your choice — cucumbers, celery, tomatoes, purple onions, sundried tomatoes, mushrooms, etc. Toss lightly with salad dressing.

Veggie Pizza

Make a crust or use a premade crust. Add pizza sauce and your favorite veggies but hold the cheese.

Veggie Calzone

Roll out frozen or fresh bread dough. Fill with your favorite cooked veggies. Roll up and seal dough so it looks like a long loaf of French bread. Place on a cookie sheet seam side down. Bake at 350 degrees for 30 to 40 minutes until golden brown. Serve with warmed pizza or marinara sauce.

Other ideas:

Soups with Noodles and Vegetables
Pita Sandwiches with Hummus and Veggies
Spaghetti with Marinara Sauce
Pasta Primavera
Black Beans on Toast or Tortilla

"D" FOODS

chicken, no skin
fish
seafood
turkey, no skin

SPICES, CONDIMENTS, AND MISCELLANEOUS

butter, light
sugar, all kinds

SNACKS

candy, sugar based, all kinds
    cinnamon bears
    gummy bears
    hard candy
    licorice
    taffy
frozen yogurt, nonfat
hot chocolate, nonfat
popcicles
sugar-based drinks, Koolaid, Gatorade, etc.

"F" FOODS

"F" stands for FAT. These foods if eaten regularly and in large quantities will make you fat and unhealthy. If you constantly "tease" yourself with these foods, your taste buds will not have a chance to be cleansed and you will have an extremely hard time making healthy food choices.

animal products
    ribs
    sausage, all kinds
    bacon
    wienies
    hamburger
    pork
    beef
    cured or salted meat or fish
butter
cakes
chocolate candy in any form
chicken with skin
cookies
eggs
dairy products
    butter
    milk
    cream
    yogurt
    cheese
duck
roasted nuts and seeds

Chapter Six

Secrets About Food That Will Change Your Life!

Diet Tips

1. If no one sees you eat it, it has no calories/fat.
2. If you drink a diet soda with a candy bar they will cancel each other out.
3. Calories/fats don't count if you eat with someone and you both eat the same amount.
4. Food taken for medicinal purposes does not count. This includes brownies, hot chocolate, brandy and Sara Lee chocolate cake.
5. If you fatten up everyone around you, you'll look thinner.
6. Snacks consumed at a movie do not count as they are part of the entertainment. For example: Milk Duds, popcorn with butter, red licorice, and M&Ms.
7. Pieces of cookies contain no calories/fat. The process of breaking causes a calorie/fat leakage.
8. Late-night snacks have no calories. The refrigerator light is not strong enough for the calories to see their way into the calorie counter.

This is one of those interoffice memos which gives us such a chuckle because it strikes so close to home. Now that you have developed a truly healthy way of eating, you can really chuckle because you realize that many of the implications in this list are just plain false. Besides, you're not operating with a "dieting" mentality anymore, and you feel and look so good, you've long forgotten about feeling guilty from eating large portions.

To help you understand and apply the Food G.P.A. to a higher level of success, I have included this additional chapter which addresses a few more food issues.

Remember:

1.   There is no such thing as "cheating" with your Food G.P.A.
2.   It's impossible to mess up with Oxycise!
3.   Listen to your body

What the heck is food combining and what's in it for me?

Just like any other part of your body, your digestive tract has certain limitations. Food combining is based on the fact that you have different types of digestive juices to break down different types of food. Protein, including all flesh foods (beef, chicken, fish, pork, lamb, or any other animal), dairy products, and nuts demand a digestive juice that is acidic in its nature. Starches such as breads, pastas, grains, potatoes, and cereals demand a digestive juice that is alkaline in nature.

Here's what happens in a typical American diet: You have a "normal" meal of meat and potatoes, fish and rice, chicken and noodles, eggs and toast, cheese and bread, or milk and cereal. The type of digestive juice secreted for the digestion of the protein food is of no value in digesting the starch food. In fact, some digestive juices cancel each other out when forced into contact with each other. The food is in your stomach for the purpose of digestion, but with the acid and alkali canceling each other out, *there are no working digestive juices to do the job.*

Undigested protein putrefies and undigested starch ferments and *no nutrients* are incorporated into healthy cell structures. Not only that, toxic acids are generated in the body. Have you ever experienced gas, flatulence, heartburn, acid indigestion, headaches, lethargy, backaches, or colds? These can be the result of inefficient digestion. *Don't you think it's strange that it has become common practice to medicate yourself after eating?*

After fueling your body, you should feel energized and ready to conquer the world. If you throw all kinds of food into your stomach at the same time, your world conquering energy dissolves into food-digesting energy and you can barely grab the remote before falling on the couch.

Food combining is essential for weight loss and general health. I started practicing these principles over 10 years ago, and I still can't believe what a difference it makes in my energy level and body comfort. Try it for one month and see for yourself.

Food Combining Made Easy

1. Eat any food within a category together with another food in the same category.

    Categories:

    A. Fruits
    B. Vegetables
    C. Starches/complex carbohydrates
    D. Proteins/meat products/dairy/nuts

2. Eat Fruits by themselves. Fruit digests very rapidly so you only need to wait about 30 minutes before eating food from other categories.

    During the Three Day Oxycise! Cleanse, you don't need to be extremely concerned with separating fruits and vegetables.

3. When eating foods from the remaining categories, combine them in the following manner.

    Starches and Vegetables Together

    ### OR

    Protein and Vegetables Together

That's all there is to remember. If you live a vegetarian lifestyle, food combining basically becomes a moot point, except for eating occasional nuts.

By the way, you may notice that there isn't a category for candy, ice cream, and other junk food. That's because you won't ever be putting that poison into your body again. Wait, wait!!! Don't throw the book away. I was just kidding. I may be idealistic, but I'm also a realist. . . . (Does that mean I'm an idealistic realist?) Anyway, the facts are that you will probably from time to time find an occasion when you choose to eat garbage. Doing it once in awhile is *"better than"* every day. So when that time comes, the best thing you can do is give your body a chance to be able to process the garbage.

Don't eat a big heavy meal and then throw down a triple scoop, hot fudge, banana split with whipped cream, nuts, and cherry on top. Instead, eat the garbage food when your stomach is empty and has the best chance of coping with the mess. My suggested time would be in the middle of the afternoon rather than in the morning (when your body is busy with elimination) or late at night (when your metabolism is slowing down and getting ready for sleeping).

Everyone I've known who has adopted food combining has been delighted with the results. Go ahead and try it. You will love how you feel!

Is eating meat really that bad?

Yes. Vegetarians suffer significantly less from all major degenerative diseases and live years longer than the rest of the population. As a group, vegetarians have been found to have lower blood pressure, more ideal blood cholesterol levels, and a generally stronger immune system. Animal protein diets are dangerous. They are a major cause of osteoporosis, kidney disease, heart disease, diabetes, arthritis, certain forms of cancer, and *obesity*.

Speaking of osteoporosis, research for over 75 years has continually shown that meat eating causes a net loss of calcium. When you consume large quantities of animal protein your blood becomes too acidic and another one of your body's set point mechanisms kicks into action. The blood, which must be maintained in a slightly alkaline state for good health, counteracts the acidity by dissolving your bones in order to provide alkaline salts to neutralize the acid. The filtration rate through your kidneys is increased, and thus the quantity of calcium lost in your urine is increased. It is impossible to keep your body in a positive calcium balance as long as you eat a lot of animal protein.

The number-one prerequisite of a food is most certainly its fuel value, fuel as it relates to energy for the body's use. Flesh foods supply *no* fuel, *no* energy. Fuel is built from carbohydrates. Meat has virtually *no* carbohydrates. In other words, **no fuel value**. What all the available evidence points to is that there is no nutritional, physiological, or psychological justification for meat-eating by humans.

It's best to stick with plant sources for protein. A varied menu of grains, beans, and vegetables contains more than enough protein for human needs. Also, there is no need to carefully combine proteins. Any variety of plant foods provides sufficient protein for your needs.

Neal Barnard, M.D., head of the Physicians Committee for Responsible Medicine advocates four new basic food groups: grains, legumes, fruits, and vegetables. According to Dr.

Barnard, "The basic dietary guidelines taught to us as children are wrong. The goal will be to get the public to recognize and accept the fact that we've turned the corner in nutrition. You don't alleviate diseases with a chicken or lean-meat diet but with a pure vegetarian diet. Research is now clear and sufficient enough to recommend this. We're not saying that you can never have another Haagen Dazs, but the basis of a healthful diet is not meat, fish, or cheese."

For a more in-depth discussion on the problems with animal protein, please go to your local library and you will find mountains of research in every medical journal and health publication. I've also included some excellent references at the end of this book that will help you with any further questions you may have. If the results of these reports don't scare you into action, then I don't know what else to do. At least, please be sure if you choose to eat meat that you combine it properly as described above so that your body is given its best chance to process it.

I was raised eating beef, elk, or venison steak for literally three meals a day, so I was a "hard sell" on this topic. It took tremendous effort for me to change my mind and habits to a vegetarian way of eating and preparing food. Besides, I thought vegetarians were a little goofy. I also worried that my husband, who was raised on a ranch in Wyoming, would have a fit if he wasn't treated with prime rib or fried chicken on a regular basis. My children had been given their share of hot dogs and hamburgers, too. And what would I serve company?

The change couldn't have been easier. I suggest doing it "cold turkey." Many times I've heard my husband say, "You know what I would love right now? A tomato sandwich on some good whole wheat bread." He loves to offer fruit smoothies to friends who stop by.

My children have a similar story. Two of them are self-declared vegetarians without any prompting from me. The other two will eat meat on occasion but have never said a word about it not being offered at home. They have all become hearty fruit and salad eaters, and it's not uncommon for my 10-year-old to pack a tomato sandwich, grapes, and a fruit drink for school lunch. I haven't had to do any preaching with them. All I did was fill the house with plenty of healthy food for snacks and mealtime. Their own bodies and taste buds did the rest. I learned that if you don't keep your family's taste buds coated with grease, meat, candy, and pop, then they will naturally choose healthy food.

But I thought milk "does a body good" . . .

Cow's milk is designed to help a baby calf double in size within six *weeks*. A human baby nourished by human milk doubles in size in six *months*. Now that you're done growing and your children are in a much slower growth period than their first six months, do you really need the milk of another species with all its saturated fat and potential disease?

In addition to the high fat and cholesterol problems, dairy products have been conclusively linked to heart attack and stroke. When milk consumption of different societies is compared, *there is a general upward trend in osteoporosis in those societies with the increased milk intake.* Surprising, but true. Casein (milk protein) has also been frequently linked to infections, allergies, bronchial infections, asthma, skin rashes, rheumatoid arthritis, and other inflammations. In fact, half the world's population is lactose intolerant. I can't imagine any of you continuing to demand this high-fat "calcium supplement" while knowing of all these common side effects.

An excuse for consuming such high amounts of dairy products has been to be sure to get enough calcium. Human beings *do* need calcium; it is an essential mineral. But all calcium comes originally from the earth. The calcium is absorbed in plants. Then animals eat the plants that contain calcium. The calcium in cow's milk comes from the plants that were eaten by the cow. This is exactly the same place where you should be getting your calcium — from plants.

Adult cows do not drink cow's milk. They do not develop weak bones because of lack of dairy products. They obtain calcium from vegetation. But more importantly, the human populations of the world who have the very best bone health consume vegetables, grains, legumes, and fruits.

It's easier than you think to have plenty of calcium in your diet. In fact, if you're eating fruits and vegetables daily and some raw nuts even occasionally, you can't have a calcium deficiency.

Here are some great sources of calcium:

alfalfa
asparagus
beans
broccoli
cabbage
carrots

cauliflower
collard greens
green leafy vegetables
lettuce
nuts, raw
onions
oranges
potatoes
rice
sesame seeds
spinach
tofu

Get rid of dairy products, even the "lite" ones, and replace them with live, healthy food without all the dangerous side effects.

You can conquer dining out!

Why is it that when you're at a restaurant or at a party you suddenly disconnect your brain and all knowledge and commitment concerning health? It wouldn't matter so much if you only went out once or twice a year, but most of you have several events every week, from casual to formal. Please keep your brain engaged and once again listen to your body as you encounter all the situations where fat, cholesterol, sugar, and chemicals are placed before you in the guise of real food. Grandma will still love you even if you don't have a piece of pie. You do not need to eat for other people. Be true to yourself.

The main key here is to be *assertive*. The second key is to be *creative*. If there is nothing listed specifically on the menu that serves your needs, ask for substitutions. Many times you can mix and match items from different menu selections or the a la carte section and end up with a wonderful meal. You'll be surprised at the willingness of chefs to create special meals for you.

Be specific in requesting that your food be cooked without any oil or butter. Leave off the melted cheese. After eating such clean food at home, it will feel disgusting to have your mouth coated with grease and you won't enjoy your evening out as much.

A wonderful bonus is how little you'll be charged for eating healthy. I've been told many times, "Oh, I can't charge you full price since you didn't have the meat."

If you are going to an event that is notorious for the poor quality of food, then eat before you go or take some food with you. If you are surprised with a poor selection of food, choose as wisely as you can or just don't eat. It's that simple. You will not die if you miss a meal or a snack. Making these extra efforts to take care of your body will ensure that you feel great at the event rather than grimacing from indigestion. You will move faster in achieving your body change goals. *And* you will help other people gain health because they will follow your example. It's worth the effort.

Yes, you are making the grade!

As you strive for Highest Honors with your Food G.P.A., remember these things:

- All food is not created equal, and different foods have different reactions in your body.

- Thin people eat more quantity and better quality food than fat people. Traditional dieting will cause you to gain weight. It is also the precursor to binging and food disorders.

- Feeding yourself or others unhealthy food is not an expression of kindness or love.

- Listen to your body and feed it as it needs fuel.

- Don't purposefully skip meals.

- Don't purposefully eat small portions.

- Eat what you truly need.

- Plant food is rich in carbohydrate and fiber. Animal products don't have them.

- Plant-based diets promote slimness. Animal products promote overweight.

Your body will thrive when given the right fuel!

May you and those you love enjoy a lifetime of health, vitality, and joy. *Here's to your health!*

BIBLIOGRAPHY

Baker, E. Oxygen: the key to energy. How diet affects oxygen intake and use. *Total Health*, Oct 1991, v13, n5, p18

Baker, E. *The Unmedical Miracle: Oxygen.* Drelwood Communications, 1991.

Barnard, N. *Eat Right, Live Longer.* Harmony Books, 1995.

Barnard, N. *Food for Life.* Harmony Books, 1993.

Barnard, N. *Foods That Cause You to Lose Weight: The Negative Calorie Effect.* Magni Company, 1992.

Covey, S. *The 7 Habits of Highly Effective People.* Simon & Schuster, New York, 1989.

Diamond, H. and M. *Fit for Life.* Warner Books, Inc., 1985

Diamond, H. and M. *Fit for Life II: Living Health.* Warner Books, Inc., 1987.

McDougall, J. *The McDougall Program. Twelve Days to Dynamic Health.* NAL Books, 1990.

McDougall, J. *McDougall's Medicine: A Challenging Second Opinion.* New Century, 1985.

Shelton, H.M. *Food Combining Made Easy.* Dr. Shelton's Health School, 1951.

Breathe deeply and eat well!

Listen to your body.

Oxycise! International, Inc. continues to consult individuals, groups and businesses who want to take control of their body weight, health,and fitness. Support materials include books, audiotapes,videotapes,and seminars.

To schedule a consultation or seminar, or to obtain additional Oxycise! System materials, write to:

Jill Johnson
Oxycise! International, Inc.
8170 S. University Blvd., #110
Littleton, CO 80122
(303)224-9588

http://www.oxycise.com